# Sexual And Reproductive Health With Nutrition And Herbs (Part I)

## Powerful Nature For Powerful Reproductive And Sexual Health

By

## Nwadiohamma Ahajumobi

Kindle Digital Publishing

**ISBN:** 9798866916979



Sexual And Reproductive Health With Nutrition And Herbs

# Sexual And Reproductive Health With Nutrition And Herbs

## TABLE OF CONTENTS (TOC)




**ISBN:** 9798866916979


# Introduction

# Sexual And Reproductive Health With Nutrition And Herbs

Millions of people from across the globe are struggling with reproduction and sexual burden. Many feel embarrassed to discuss these problems with anyone or physicians. To me, the problem is there for human beings to fix them. I share in your burden and I am here to break the ice that we may start from someone on a journey to tackle the sexual and reproductive illnesses through simple nutrition and herbal approaches, which may not break the bank to fix. Today, I came with good news from nutrition and herbs so, I ask you to calm down, read and explore and you will be glad that you did.

Sexual And Reproductive Health With Nutrition And Herbs

Sexual dysfunction is a common occurrence in the lives of many people, especially men over 40 years of age. In the United States, over 60% of women and nearly 60% of men experience sexual dysfunction. The problem is not unique to the United States, as Sub-Saharan Africa also faces high rates of sexual problems, particularly among individuals with diabetes in Nigeria. By 2025, it is estimated that as many as 322 million men worldwide will be affected by sexual problems. However, these figures may be underestimated due to the stigma attached to discussing sexual issues (5, 9, 10, 11).

Sexual And Reproductive Health With Nutrition And Herbs

Since sexual dysfunction is a global epidemic that occurs at some point in someone's life at adulthood, providing education and creating awareness through a powerful electronic medium such as Kindle Digital Publishing becomes very handy in getting the message across to global communities. Because the existing sexual dysfunction treatments are insufficient and often, side and adverse effects underscore the benefits.

Sexual And Reproductive Health With Nutrition And Herbs

# Chapter I. Causes of Sexual Dysfunction

It's worth noting that millions of couples silently struggle with sexual dysfunction. Many dare not to mention or discuss reproductive or sexual illnesses often, due to feelings of shame or embarrassment, which prevent them from discussing their issues with healthcare professionals or even with each other (5, 6).

New findings in the field of reproductive and sexual health have identified connections with nutrition and herbal remedies. Scientific research has indicated that sexual

Sexual And Reproductive Health With Nutrition And Herbs

dysfunction can be linked to a number of factors namely:

1. Cell oxidation and lipid peroxidation

2. Hypoxia

3. Low sex hormones

4. Low levels of sex hormones

5. Enzymes

1. Cell Oxidation and lipid Peroxidation

Lipids are fats and oil. Consuming too much is injurious to health and consuming unhealthy lipids is even worse. Consume moderate

Sexual And Reproductive Health With Nutrition And Herbs

amounts of healthy lipids and avoid unhealthy lipids consumption. Peroxidation is oxidation process that involves chain of reaction of bad or degraded lipids, mainly polyunsaturated lipids to form a harmful compound called free radical, which is injurious to reproductive health. Free radicals forcefully take electrons from lipids inside the cell membrane to cause harm to the cell. Peroxides are formed from lipids oxidation when two atoms of oxygen is involve, but when only one atom of oxygen is involved, the product is simply oxide of the lipids or lips oxidation.

This underscores the importance of the oils that enter the body Sexual And Reproductive Health With Nutrition And Herbs through daily consumption. Whether fats or oil get into the body directly as dietary oils or through foods prepared with these oils, it affects sexual function, re-productive health and overall well-being. Olive, avocado and original fresh and unadulterated palm oil and moderate consumption of co-conut oil are good sources. Trans fatty acid, and polyunsaturated fats and oils are

highly injurious to health and ad-versely affects a person's repro-ductive and sex health (1, 2, 3, 4, 5).

## 2. Cell oxidation
High intake of unhealthy lipids

Sexual And Reproductive Health With Nutrition And Herbs

cause rise in the amount of reactive oxygen species, which cause cell oxidation or decay. Cell oxidation opens doors of chronic diseases including reproductive and sexual disorders. Also lack of essential nutrients, minerals and vitamins for a prolonged period of time also add up to cell oxidation (1, 2, 3, 4, 5).

3. Hypoxia

Another significant factor impacting sexual health is the extended periods of low oxygen levels in cells, known as hypoxia. Conditions like obesity, diabetes, and cardiovascular diseases can lead to relaxed arteries in the penis when they should be erect, which

Sexual And Reproductive Health With Nutrition And Herbs

inhibits the production of nitric oxide, a crucial factor for natural and desirable penile erection. Moreover, diets rich in unhealthy fats can contribute to the production of harmful reactive oxygen species (13, 14, 15, 16).

## 4. Low Levels of Sex Hormones

Low levels of sex hormones such as estrogen, progesterone, and testosterone, can lead to unsatisfactory sexual performance and in some cases cause reproductive problems. Prolonged deficiencies in vitamins E and A, as well as low zinc levels, can also contribute to reduced sex hormone levels. Additionally, elevated levels of reactive metals such as calcium ions

(Ca2+) can further decrease the amounts of estrogen, progesterone, and testosterone. Vitamins E and A are effective antioxidants which protects the body from cell oxidation, reinforces body immunity and keeps the body safe from chronic diseases and sexual dysfunction. Vitamins E and A are essential for female and male reproductive health. Vitamin A is important for eye health and growth (1, 2, 3, 4, 5, 6, 7, 12).

## 5. Enzymes

Specific enzymes do harm to sexual organs. Certain enzymes can negatively influence sexual performance. Examples of enzymes

Sexual And Reproductive Health With Nutrition And Herbs

linked to poor sexuality include-Arginase, phosphodiesterase-5 (PDE-5), and Acetylcholinesterase (AchE). On the other hand, Angiotensin-converting enzymes play a crucial role in penile erection.

Sexual And Reproductive Health With Nutrition And Herbs

Chapter II. Types of Sexual dysfunction

There are various categories of sexual dysfunction, which include the disorders related to:

a. Lack of desire
b. Poor arousal
c. Unsatisfactory orgasms,
d. Poor coupling or mounting
e. Poor intromission or penetration
f. Weak erection
g. Delayed latency
h. Low sperm count
I. Weak egg and poor ovulation
j. Sexual pain disorders
k. Painful menstruation

All these are forms of sexual disorders or reproductive problems, Sexual And Reproductive Health With Nutrition And Herbs

which can affect someone's sex
life or relationship negatively. Because sex and relationships are vi-
tal aspects of human life, this is a
good ground to take action to address the problem.

Sexual And Reproductive Health With
Nutrition And Herbs

# Chapter III. Environmental Causes of Reproductive Disorders

The causes of some of these disorders can be diverse and may include psychological factors like such as;

1. Anxiety and Stress

2. Chronic diseases

3. Neurological diseases like Alzheimer's and Parkinson's diseases,
   spinal cord and nerve injuries

4. Lifestyle factors such as substance abuse, and long-term usage of

drugs to treat the previously mentioned conditions (6).

Several factors can impact human sexuality. Stress, for instance, triggers oxidative stress in the body, leading to the release of cortisol. Stress hormones can suppress sex hormones and sexual desires, affecting libido, sexual activity, and fertility.

## 1. Anxiety And Stress

High levels of stress and anxiety also have adverse effects on females, affecting fertilization, implantation of fertilized eggs, and pregnancy retention. When people experience a feeling of stress, oxidative stress is in action, and the human body responds to it by the release of stress hormones called cortisol, which suppresses sex hormones-gametes, and sex desires and frequency to have sex namely, libido, sexual intercourse, and fertility problems. For females it affects the fertilization, implantation of fertilized egg, and pregnancy retention. The wistar rats used for this experiment showed significant reduction of their cortisol levels after the experiment.

## 2. Chronic Disease

A chunk of people with sexual dysfunction have one chronic disease or another. Sexual dysfunction is

Sexual And Reproductive Health With Nutrition And Herbs

not unique to the United States, as Sub- Saharan Africa also faces high rates of sexual problems, particularly among individuals with diabetes in Nigeria. It is the same with high blood pressure (3, 4, 5, 6).

## 3. Neurological Diseases

A good amount of people with neurological diseases like Alzheimer's and Parkinson's diseases, spinal cord and nerve injuries experience a form of reproductive problem or the other.

## 4. Lifestyle Factors

Lifestyle factors such as substance abuse, and long-term usage of

Sexual And Reproductive Health With Nutrition And Herbs

drugs to treat some chronic conditions show adversity to a person's
sexual life (6).

Sexual And Reproductive Health With
Nutrition And Herbs

# Chapter IV. Herbal Products with Effective Sexual Health

In the quest to address sexual dysfunction and reproductive health issues naturally, many plant-based products and remedies have emerged as effective solutions.

Some plant extracts, like those from dates, coconut, and tiger nuts, have shown the ability to inhibit the harmful effects of enzymes like phosphodiesterase-5 and Arginases, thereby promoting better penile erection. This beneficial effect is attributed to the high levels of phytochemical compounds, such as flavonoids, found in these extracts (1, 3, 6, 14, 15, 16, 17, 18).

One such example is "Kunu Aya," a beverage made from a blend of tiger nuts, coconut milk, and dates. 'Kunu Aya' is originally a popular refreshing drink in Nigeria's major cities, this drink has been found to have powerful sexual enhancing effects. It boosts testosterone levels, positively influences mood, and inhibits factors associated with erectile dysfunction.

In a research study to determine the effect and mechanism of these nuts' extracts ('Kunu Aya') effect on aphrodisiac and fertility enhancement. The in vivo tested ex-

Sexual And Reproductive Health With Nutrition And Herbs

periment with Wistar rats to perform the test for aphrodisiac and fertility capabilities of extract of each nut and the blend of the extracts in comparison with the control and standard sexual enhancement medication, sildenafil.

The effect of use of 'Kunu Aya' on the behaviours and physical characteristics of tested animals such as frequency of mounting and mating, biochemical factors namely, sperm count, prostate specific antigen, testosterone as well as the psychological or anxiolytic effect such as mood. The results showed that the individual nut extract and a blend of the three nuts namely dates, coconut and Tiger

Sexual And Reproductive Health With Nutrition And Herbs

nuts- 'Kunu- Aya' showed ability to improve sexual and reproductive behaviour. The results revealed a significant frequency of mating, sexual arousal, motivation, vigour and

sexual intercourse compared with standard medication for treating sexual arousal such as sildenafil. The reality of reproductive and sexual problems in today's world is a significant concern for overall wellness and procreation. Nobody wants to face difficulties in their sex life or have their relationships strained due to sexual problems. While medical treatments are available, they can be expensive and come with side effects. Herbal Sexual And Reproductive Health With Nutrition And Herbs solutions continue to show promise for effectively managing sexual dysfunction (4, 5, 6).

In summary, the research discussed in this book sheds light on the powerful potential of nutrition and plant-based products for managing sexual dysfunction and improvement of reproductive health. Alternative solutions with little or no adverse effect offer hope for individuals seeking effective and affordable options to enhance sexual well-being and overall quality of life.

A brief summaries of various herbs from different parts of the world used for reproductive purposes

Sexual And Reproductive Health With Nutrition And Herbs

with a highlight on their rich phyto-chemical compounds, which are responsible for their effectiveness in traditional use for sexual dysfunction will be discussed in the part II of the series.

## Reference

Sexual And Reproductive Health With Nutrition And Herbs

5.Ahajumobi, E. N., & Anderson, P. B. (2022). Hunteria Umbellata Extract is a Potent Agent for EffecTive Diabetes Control. Asian Journal of Medicine and Health, 20(8), 26-36. https://doi.org/ 10.9734/ajmah/2022/ v20i830479

6.Ahajumobi, E. N. (2022) Nutrients, Vitamins, Mineral and Hydration for Health Restoration. iUniverse, Liberty Drive Bloomington, IN 47403. ISBN: 9781663237408 https://www.iuniverse.com/en/ bookstore

7.Constance Tom Noguchi and Alan N. Inhibition of sickle hemoglobin gelation by amino acids and related compounds. Schechter

Sexual And Reproductive Health With Nutrition And Herbs

Biochemistry 1978 17 (25), 5455-5459. DOI: 10.1021/ bi00618a020

8.Ajayi, Ibironke A., and Olusola O. Ojelere. "Chemical composition of ten medicinal plant seeds from Southwest Nigeria." Advances in Life Science and Technology 10 (2013): 25-32.

9.Ahajumobi, N. E., Oparaocha, T. E. A Comparative Analysis of Nutritional and Chemical composition of Seven Leaves Used as Folk Medicine in South Eastern Nigeria. International Journal of Recent Advances in Multidisciplinary Research. 2023; 10(8): 8763-8773. http:// www.ijramr.com/issue/com-

Sexual And Reproductive Health With Nutrition And Herbs

parative-analysis-nutritional-and-chemical- composition-seven-leaves-used-folk-medicine

10. Ahajumobi, E. N., & Anderson, P. B. (2023). Hunteria Umbellata for Aphrodisiac Therapy. International Journal of Innovation Scientific Research and Review. 2023, 5(4): 4324-4329. ISSN: 2582-6131. http:// journalijisr.com/ issue/hunteria-umbellata-aphrodisiac-therapy

11. Ahajumobi, E. N. (2022) Nutrients, Vitamins, Mineral and Hydration for Health Restoration. iUniverse, Liberty Drive Bloomington, IN 47403. ISBN: 9781663237408

Sexual And Reproductive Health With Nutrition And Herbs

https://www.iuniverse.com/en/bookstore

12.Olaniyan, Olugbemi Tope, Olufadekemi Tolulope Kunle-Alabi, and Yinusa Raji. "Protective effects of methanol extract of Plukenetia conophora seeds and 4H-Pyran-4-One 2, 3-Dihydro-3, 5-Dihydroxy-6-

Methyl on the reproductive function of male Wistar rats treated with

cadmium chloride." JBRA assisted reproduction 22.4 (2018): 289.

13.Erhenhi, A. H., and B. O. Obadoni. "Known medicinal and aphrodisiac plants of Urhonigbe

Sexual And Reproductive Health With Nutrition And Herbs

forest reserve, Edo State, Nigeria." J Med Plants

Stud 3.4 (2015): 101-6.

14.Oseyomon, J. O., and E. E. Ilodigwe. "Toxicological evaluation of

methanol seed extract of hunteria umbellata on reproductive functions of treated wistar rats." African Journal of Health, Safety and Environment 2.2 (2021): 71-88.

15.Kadiri, M., A. W. Ojewumi, and T. N. Onatade. "Indigenous uses and phytochemical contents of plants used in the treatment of menstrual disorders and after-child birth problems in abeokuta south local government area of Ogun Sexual And Reproductive Health With Nutrition And Herbs

State, Nigeria." Journal of Drug Delivery and Therapeutics (2015): 33-42.

16.Oboh, Ganiyu, Adeniyi A. Adebayo, and Ayokunle O. Ademosun. "Erection-stimulating, anti-diabetic and antioxidant properties of Hunteria umbellata and Cylicodiscus gabunensis water extractable phytochemicals." Journal of Complementary and Integrative Medicine 15.1 (2018).

17.Goel, Bharti, and Neelesh Kumar Maurya. "Aphrodisiac Herbal therapy for Erectile Dysfunction." Archives of Pharmacy Practice 11.1 (2020).

Sexual And Reproductive Health With Nutrition And Herbs

18.Prieto, Dolores, et al. "Hypoxic relaxation of penile arteries: involvement of endothelial nitric oxide and modulation by reactive oxygen species." American Journal of Physiology-Heart and Circulatory Physiology 299.3 (2010): H915-H924.

19.Prieto, Dolores, et al. "Hypoxic relaxation of penile arteries: involvement of endothelial nitric oxide and modulation by reactive oxygen species." American Journal of Physiology-Heart and Circulatory Physiology 299.3 (2010): H915-H924.

20.Oboh, Ganiyu, et al. "In vitro inhibition of phosphodiesterase-5 and arginase activities from rat penile tissue by two Nigerian herbs (Hunteria umbellata and Anogeissus leiocarpus)." Journal of basic and clinical physiology and pharmacology 28.4 (2017): 393-401.

21.Oboh, Ganiyu, et al. "Aphrodisiac effect of Hunteria umbellata seed extract: Modulation of nitric oxide level and arginase activity in vivo." Pathophysiology 26.1 (2019): 39-47.

22.Oboh, Ganiyu, Adeniyi A. Adebayo, and Ayokunle O. Ademosun. "Erection-stimulating, anti-diabetic and antioxidant properties of Hunteria umbellata and Cylicodiscus gabunensis water extractable phytochemicals." Journal of Complementary and Integrative Medicine 15.1 (2018).

ISBN: 9798866916979


Sexual And Reproductive Health With Nutrition And Herbs

www.ingramcontent.com/pod-product-compliance
Lightning Source LLC
Chambersburg PA
CBHW070753260726
48660CB00007B/3092